Mara Simoncini
Sabrina D'Agostino
Antonia Gatti Piero Ettore Quirico

Acupressure in insomnia for patients with Alzheimer's disease

Mara Simoncini
Sabrina D'Agostino
Antonia Gatti Piero Ettore Quirico

Acupressure in insomnia for patients with Alzheimer's disease

LAP LAMBERT Academic Publishing

Cover image: www.ingimage.com

Publisher:
LAP LAMBERT Academic Publishing
is a trademark of
Dodo Books Indian Ocean Ltd. and OmniScriptum S.R.L publishing group

120 High Road, East Finchley, London, N2 9ED, United Kingdom
Str. Armeneasca 28/1, office 1, Chisinau MD-2012, Republic of Moldova, Europe
Managing Directors: Ieva Konstantinova, Victoria Ursu
info@omniscriptum.com

Printed at: see last page
ISBN: 978-3-659-62410-0

Authors

Mara Simoncini (MD, PhD)
Sabrina D'Agostino (MD)
Piero Ettore Quirico (MD)
Antonia Gatti (MD)
Silvia Balla (Psych)
Barbara Capellero (Psych)
Rossella Obialero (MD, PhD)
Nicholas Sandri (Medical Student)
Luigi Maria Pernigotti (MD)

To my parents.

We thank all those who made this project possible.

In particular, all the authors who have contributed to writing the book.

We thank the LAP for the wonderful opportunity and professionalism in their work.

We thank the KCS CAREGIVER, cooperative that manages the Nursing Homes in which our study was conducted, for the organization and management support.

We thank the Consulteam which provided free devices used.

Summary :

1.   Acupuncture, Acupressure and Traditional Chinese Medicine   pag.   9
2.   Aging in Traditional Chinese Medicine   pag. 11
3.   Dementia in Traditional Chinese Medicine   pag. 12
4.   The *Heart* and the *Shen* in Traditional Chinese Medicine   pag. 14
5.   Insomnia and anxiety-depressive symptoms in
      Traditional Chinese Medicine   pag. 17
6.   Description of the point HT 7 *Shenmen* according to
      Western Medicine and Traditional Chinese Medicine   pag. 19
7.   The efficacy of acupressure for insomnia and other
      sleep disorders in institutionalized elderly with dementia   pag. 22
      Objectives   pag. 22
         I.   Mini Mental State Examination (MMSE)   pag. 22
         II.   Global Deterioration Scale (GDS)   pag. 24
         III.   Neuropsychiatric Inventory (NPI)   pag. 26
         IV.   General Health Questionnaire 28 (GHQ 28)   pag. 28
         V.   State Trait Anxiety Inventory Y-1 (STAY)   pag. 29
         VI.   Pittsburg Sleep Quality Index (PSQI)   pag. 30
         VII.   Activity of Daily Living (ADL)   pag. 31
         VIII.   Instrumental Activity of Daily Living (IADL)   pag. 31
      Methods   pag. 32
      Results   pag. 36
      Discussion   pag. 41
      Conclusions   pag. 43
8.   References   pag. 44

1. Acupuncture, Acupressure and Traditional Chinese Medicine

The origin of acupuncture is remote: some historical sources report that already 3,000 / 4,000 years ago in ancient China a rudimentary acupuncture was practiced with needles made of bone or metals. Other sources also reported that a massage in certain sections of the body was practiced for therapeutic purposes.

The oldest text regarding acupuncture that surviving until today is the *Suwen Neijing* (Canon of Internal Medicine of Emperor *Huang Di*) which dates back to the second century A.C.

The discovery of acupoints was random, because accidental trauma or self-massage of aching zones were able to alleviate the pain or also solve particular problems.

Acupoints, subsequently grouped into *Channels* or *Meridians*, became an important therapeutic tool for Chinese Medicine and formed the basis of two major disciplines: **Acupuncture** and **Massage**.

Scientific experiments have shown that the mechanisms of acupuncture's action may involve simple segmental nerve reflexes, but also complex mesencephalic and diencephalic circuits.

The main effects of acupuncture described by various authors are the following:

- Trophic effect, that regulates blood flow in different parts of the body and restore proper tissue trophism;

- Anti-inflammatory effect and regulation of the immune system, that is useful for the resolution of inflammatory diseases;

- Analgesic effect at three levels: spinal cord, mesencephalic and pituitary, through the secretion of neurotransmitters (dynorphins, enkephalins, catecholamines, endorphins);

- Antispasmodic effect that causes somatic and visceral musculature relaxation, very useful in the treatment of many painful conditions (acute low back pain, abdominal colic...);

- Anxiolytic and antidepressant effects with action on limbic system and cerebral cortex and on the regulation of secretion of several neuromediators (endorphins, serotonin, GABA, etc.) involved in various mental processes;

- Neuro-hormonal regulation of the hypothalamic-pituitary-gonadal axis and other endocrine mechanisms which enable control of homeostasis *(1, 2, 3, 4)*.

The combination of these effects makes it possible to treat several diseases, algic and not, by acting on pathogenetic mechanisms.

The main treatments used in Traditional Chinese Medicine are :

1) **Acupuncture** that uses needles in particular body sites (acupoints) for therapeutic purposes;

2) **Electro-acupuncture** with electrical acupoint stimulation;

3) **Cupping therapy** which consists of applying cups on acupoint;

4) **Bleeding** in order to renew the circulation;

5) **Moxibustion** that consists in thermic acupoint stimulation by cigars of mugwort;

6) **Acupressure** that consists in acupoint massage for a necessary time.

Acupressure is based on the same principles as acupuncture and consists in a massage or a stimulation of some acupuncture points, performed without needles, reproducing an effect usually defined as ''needle sensation'' or ''*De Qi*'' *(5, 6, 7)*.

Acupressure does not only relax the human body; it also stimulates the physiological functions of acupuncture channels. Therefore, acupressure can promote health and offer comfort in several diseases *(8, 9)*.

Additionally, acupressure is more effective especially as regards tolerability. It allows to treat safely elderly patients for agitation, insomnia and pain with positive results and without drugs' side effects.

Furthermore acupressure can be associated with western therapies with positive results *(10, 11)*.

2. Aging in Traditional Chinese Medicine

Aging is considered a normal process, and when it evolves in a regular way is not to be considered as a disease. If the decline is slow and harmonious, brain function and functional skills are better preserved; if decline occurs in a rapid way, disorders and diseases could develop .

"Aging" in Chinese is **lǎohuà :**

老化

With age the *Qi* and the *Blood* (according to Traditional Chinese Medicine) decline after 35 years old. Around 70-80% of the elderly, has a *Qi* deficiency with *Blood stasis*. The *Qi* drives and governs the *Blood*, which is the mother of *Qi*. If *Blood* stagnates does not reach the tissues that are damaged because of this lack of *Blood*. Aging and chronic diseases damage the microcirculation and the risk of chronic diseases may be connected also to decline of immune system. This mechanism creates a vicious cycle because it worsens the circulation of *Qi* and *Blood*, and if the circulation through the *Channels* stops, the organs receive less *Blood* and *Qi*.

The decline should be slow and progressive. Premature aging can result from weakness in the *Kidney-Jing*. A gradual decline of *Kidney* will affect the various systems of the body, inducing different ways of growing old.

Acupuncture can increase the *Jing*, supporting the body in its process of aging. Acupuncture, in effect, acts on the immune system by attenuating oxidative stress and promoting the proliferation of T lymphocytes *(12)*. It is also useful the use of moxibustion that warms the acupoints and stimulates the circulation; it is known that the use of moxibustion on *GV14 (Zuhui)*, *ST36 (Zusanli)*, *BL23 (Shenshu)* and *SP6 (Sanyinjiao)* stimulates the immune system.

3. Dementia in Traditional Chinese Medicine

Among disorders related to aging, there are anxiety-depressive syndrome, memory deficits, dementia and behavior disorders including insomnia.

Dementia is a highly debilitating condition with an increasing trend in relation to the progressive aging of the population; so, it will represent one of the most important public health emergencies in the years to come. The efficiency of mental status is one of the most important aspects to maintaining the quality of life in elderly people. In most cases, the age-related modifications, such as a slowdown in learning processes or a reduction in execution speed of some cognitive tests, do not have a significant functional impact (13). When the decline of cognitive function becomes severe enough to interfere with usual social activities and work of the elderly we can talk about dementia.

Alzheimer's disease is a neurodegenerative disorder characterized by impairment of memory, abstract thinking, judgment and by changes of personality and behavior (14). We can consider Mild Cognitive Impairment (MCI) as a prodromic state of Alzheimer's disease referring to a condition between normal brain aging and the real Alzheimer's dementia. Patients with MCI usually show a loss of memory greater than what is expected for age, but at the same time does not meet the criteria for Alzheimer's disease (15). However, it is reported that the MCI has a high risk of progression to Alzheimer's disease in 10-15% (16).

The term "behavioral disorders" refers to a widely different events. According to the Consensus Conference of the International Psychogeriatric Association, The term "behavioral disorders" should be replaced by the term "Behavioral and Psychological Symptoms of Dementia" (BPSD) described as a combination of symptoms characterized by alteration of perception, content of thought, mood and behavior, that occur frequently in patients with dementia (17). The behavioral disorders can be divided into two categories: psychological disorders (delirium, hallucinations, paranoid syndrome, depression and anxiety) and behavioral disorders (physical and verbal aggression, wandering, sleep disturbance and inappropriate eating and sexual behavior).

Dementia, in Traditional Chinese Medicine, is included in the "follies" (*Dian, Kuang*), disorders marked by serious anomalies of the "mental" status (*Shen*) with prevalent alterations of the *Yin* (quiet forms, *Dian*) or of the *Yang* (agitated forms,

Kuang). In the first case, we can have apathy and depression, while in the second case, there could be agitation and irritability.

Moreover, according to Traditional Chinese Medicine (TCM), dementia does not represent only a mental disorder, because it is related to the dysfunction of some internal organs (*Zang Fu*), in particular of the *Heart*. The stimulation of specific acupoints that regulate the following five organs, *Liver, Heart, Spleen, Lung,* and *Kidney*, could decrease memory impairment *(18)*. Infact, in case of long-term memory loss, appearance of delusional ideation and agitation, we can think about a progressive emptying of the *Yin* of the *Heart*.

Acupressure could decrease agitated behaviors in patients with dementia *(19)*. Several studies show that daily acupressure treatment is effective in decreasing agitated behaviors associated with dementia and they also highlight that, using a combination of Traditional Chinese Medicine and Western medicine, as well as acupressure, agitated behaviors could decrease in patients with dementia *(20, 21)*.

In particular, in Traditional Chinese Medicine the use of *HT7* point (*Shenmen*) has clinical indication in psycho-emotional disorders, as in the treatment of anxiety, depression and, insomnia. Anxiolytic and antidepressant effects are due to a positive action on the limbic system and on cerebral cortex. In addition, the *HT7* point stimulation regulates the secretion of several neuromodulators (endorphins, serotonin, GABA, etc.), and, in particular, melatonin *(22, 1)*.

The results of a recent study indicate that intradermal *HT7* (*Shenmen*) and *PC6* (*Neiguan*) acupuncture is a useful therapeutic method against post stroke-onset insomnia, as it stabilizes and reduces the sympathetic hyperactivity *(23)*.

A recent study has clarified the mechanism of acupuncture in treating MCI and Alzheimer's disease using functional magnetic resonance imaging (fRM). They found that, compared them with healthy controls, acupuncture at *LV3* (*Taichong*) and *LI4* (*Hegu*) can activate some regions correlated with both cognition in patients with Alzheimer's disease and with Mild Cognitive Impairment (MCI) *(24)*.

So, acupuncture may be helpful in treating behavioral disorders associated with dementia, especially for agitated behavior.

4.   Insomnia and anxiety-depressive symptoms in Traditional Chinese Medicine

According to Traditional Chinese Medicine, humans have made by 2 parts, the *yin* aspect that is most physical and structural, corresponding to the body, and the *yang* aspect more ethereal, functional and dynamic, that corresponds to the mind. Every human has a more *yin* or a more *yang* aspect, but in any case the two components are indivisible. In Traditional Chinese Medicine, organs have both a mental and a physical part. Food is the feeding for the body, emotions are the nourishment for the mind. How the digestive system digests food, also mind has to "digest" emotions and then empty them out. If mind is full, it cannot accept new experiences.

The positive effect of acupuncture in the treatment of anxious-depressive syndromes has a neurophysiological substrate.

For example, a study was done on newborn rats that were taken away from mom who expressed anxious behaviors when exposed to stressful events. Their anxious behaviors were soften when treated with acupuncture on HT7 and ST36. This was caused by a modulation of neuropeptyde Y secretion in amygdala *(2)*.

Besides, electro-acupuncture on GV20 and ST36 causes a reduction of IL-1 beta and IL-6, improving depressive symptoms *(25)*.

Acupuncture combined with low doses of fluoxetine was as effective as the full dose of fluoxetine and those who had severe symptoms of anxiety and/or intolerable side effects from the drug, derived benefit from acupuncture alone *(26)*.

In a recent article, furthermore, acupuncture associated with counselling in the early stages of depressive syndromes allows to have better results after three months than patients treated with only antidepressant therapy *(27)*.

The effectiveness of acupuncture is also seen in post-stroke depression with much less side effects compared with conventional medical therapy *(28, 29)*.

Analyzing the Cochrane Database, meta-analysis and reviews on the use of acupuncture for anxious and depressive symptoms, the efficacy must be proven and data need further confirmations. They all agree, however, on the safety of the treatment and the absence of side effects *(30, 31)*.

Sleep disorders are very common in the elderly. During the last decades of life, changes in sleep quality are almost always negative in nature, and these often cause distress, mood disturbances, and an overall decline in the quality of life. In fact, while aging, sleep structure changes continuously and in a consistent way. From infancy to old age, there are marked changes in how sleep starts and continues, in its duration, in the amount of time spent in each stage of sleep, and in the overall sleep efficiency. The causes of decreased sleep efficiency are complex and rather poorly understood, but the consequences of reduced correct sleep are relatively well described.

Insomnia is characterized by one or more of the following disorders: difficulty in starting or maintaining sleep, waking up too early in the morning, and chronically non - restorative sleep or poor sleep quality. In addition, these complaints could be present despite adequate circumstances and opportunities of sleep and they could cause a reduction of daytime activities (e.g., mood disturbances, attention and memory impairments, and fatigue). Elderly with insomnia more often show symptoms like poor sleep maintenance rather than problems with sleep initiation, and the symptoms are more prevalent in those suffering also from depression, respiratory symptoms, and physical disability *(32)*.

Epidemiological studies show that approximately 50 % of all old adults suffer from significant sleep disturbances. The fact that the remaining half doesn't complain about sleep disturbances, suggests that aging per se is not necessarily related to a greater development of more sleep disorders.

Insomnia can be divided into primary or secondary one. When insomnia is not due to medical, psychiatric, or medication-related disorders, it is considered to be primary in nature *(33)*. It is estimated that primary insomnia is about 25 % of all cases of chronic insomnia. Secondary insomnia is more prevalent than primary insomnia and includes sleep disorders associated with other medical, psychiatric, or medication-related disorders such as pain syndromes, neurological disorders (e.g., dementia and Parkinson's disease), and pulmonary and cardiac disorders.

Insomnia is the most frequent clinical problem in institutionalized old patients, especially when other psychological and behavioral disturbances are also present. In some patients, pharmacological treatment could create tolerance or it could be ineffective. In addition, the pharmacological treatment is not free of side effects. Interventions for agitated behaviors are a key problem for caregivers and nursing staff, taking care of patients affected by dementia *(34, 35)*. In these patients, agitated behaviors increase the costs of formal care such as outpatient department visits, institutionalization, and inappropriate admission to the hospital.

Besides pharmacological treatments, alternative methods are frequently used, such as acupuncture and acupressure *(5, 6)*. In fact, complementary medicine for the treatment of sleep disorders has been increasingly studied over the past two decades.

Recently, in a systematic review there was a clear support in the treatment of chronic insomnia for acupressure, tai chi, yoga *(36)*. Also, another systematic review showed a beneficial effect of acupuncture compared with no treatment and with sham acupuncture on total score of Pittsburgh Sleep Quality Index (PSQI) with no serious side effects *(37)*.

Also with regard to insomnia, there is ample evidence in the literature on the efficacy of acupuncture, electro-acupuncture and auricular-acupuncture therapy. It is seen, for example, that the electro-acupuncture in primary insomnia is the most effective in the short term than the pacebo *(38)*.

In another recent study, acupuncture (associated with *sham-acupuncture*), after 6 weeks, is more effective on primary insomnia than the use of estazolam *(39)*. Also the auricular acupuncture seems effective in enhancing the quality and quantity of sleep *(40)*.

5. The *Heart* and the *Shen* in Traditional Chinese Medicine

The *Heart Channel* has 3 branches all of which begin in the heart (anatomical organ). A branch descends through the diaphragm, connecting with the small intestine. Another branch salt passing close to the trachea and reaching the eye. The third branch passes through the lung and emerges in the armpit. The *Heart Channel* crosses the median line of the inner face of the arm, elbow and forearm. It passes through the wrist and the palm of the hand and terminates on the inner side of the tip of the little finger where it connects with the *Small Intestine Channel (41)*. This is the main pathway of the *Heart Channel*.

The *Heart Channel* includes 9 acupoints (*HT1, HT2, HT3, HT4, HT5, HT6, HT7, HT8, HT9*) *(42)*

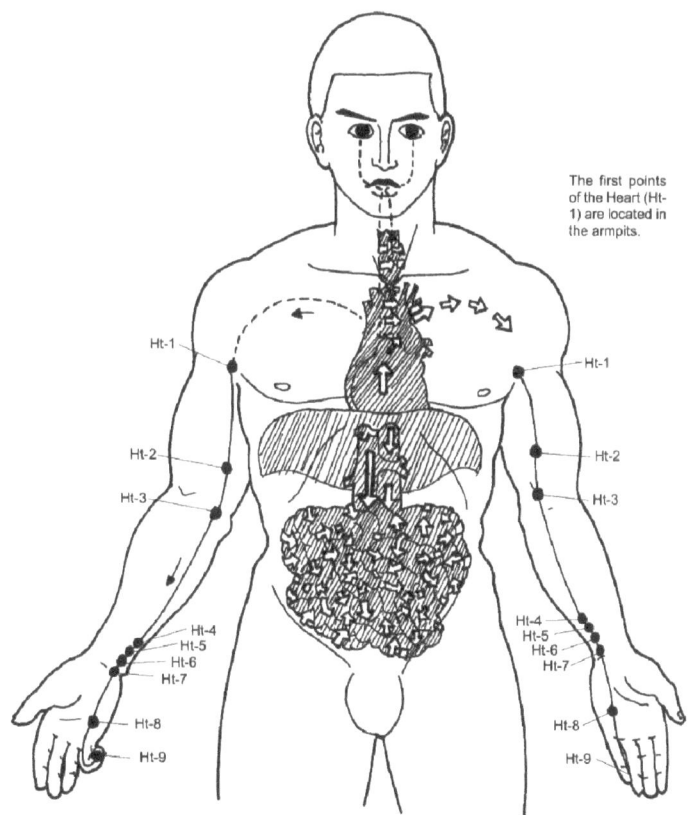

The first points of the Heart (Ht-1) are located in the armpits.

The Internal and External Qi Flow of the Heart (Ht) Channels

The *Heart* is considered the most important of all internal organs.
The functions of the *Heart* are :

1.   govern the blood, ensuring an adequate intake of blood to all organs;
2.   control the blood vessels, ensuring an full and smooth pulse;
3.   control the perspiration;
4.   the *Heart* is manifested on the tongue;
5.   the *Heart* is related to happiness;
6.   and, most important for our discussion, the *Heart* is the residence of the mind (*Shen*) and intellect which are expressed through the intensity of the eyes.

In Traditional Chinese Medicine, the *Shen* has mainly two meanings : the first includes the mental faculties and in this sense the *Shen* corresponds to the mind. Second, the *Shen* denotes the whole emotional, mental and spiritual health of the individual. In this case the *Shen* is also connected to other organs such as the *Lung* (*Pò*), the *Liver* (*Hun*), the *Spleen* (*Yi*) and the *Kidneys* (*Zhì*). *Pò, Hun, Yi, Zhì* and *Shen* represent the 5 spiritual components of the psyche.

A healthy *Shen* must be able to read the emotions as nourishment, keeping what is needed and eliminating what is not necessary. The *Liver* is the organ that filters out all the emotions. When the *Liver* is obstructed, the *Shen* is disturbed because it is clouded by his emotions. The components of the psyche are 5 and they are domiciled in various organs.

The *Pò* is the psychic entity related to the *Lung*. It is the most instinctual part of the mind, it is the mental part that pushes man by instinct to breathe, to seek nourishment, to reproduce, it is the force of instinct.

The *Hun* is related to the *Liver* and it corresponds to the soul that enters the body at birth.

The *Yi* is connected to the S*pleen* and is the ability to remember.

The *Zhì*, instead, is connected to the *Kidney* and expresses the will power.

The *Shen* collects and combines *Hun, Pò, Yi* and *Zhì*. The *Shen* can be blocked (endogenous depression), unstable (anxious-depressive syndrome with high anxiety and insomnia), weakened (anxious-depressive syndrome with low anxiety and mild or medium depression). The anxious-depressive symptoms can be traced to conditions "full" and to conditions "empty". In the elderly are mainly present latter *(43)*.

6. Description of the point *HT 7 Shenmen* according to Western and Traditional Chinese Medicine

Name: *Shenmen*

Meaning: Mind gate

神   ***Shén*** = mind, spirit, consciousness

門   ***Mèn*** = gate, door, passage

Location: on the skin crease of the wrist, between the pisiform and the ulna bones, in the medial depression of the tendon of the flexor carpis ulnaris muscle.

Posture: patient with the palm facing up.

Needling method: perpendicular.

Depth: 0.5-1 cun (0,5-1 cm)

Needle and pressure sensation (*De Qi*): local numbness and pain, possibly radiating to the ulnar aspect of the forearm and to the hand.

Moxibustion: cones 3-5; stick 5 to 10 minutes.

Anatomy: the needle crosses the skin, the subcutaneous tissue - and passing medially to the tendon of the flexor carpis ulnaris muscle - gets to the external edge of the ulnar vessel-nerve trunk.

In the superficial layer there is the anterior branch of the medial antebrachial cutaneous nerve (C8) and the palmar branch of the ulnar nerve (C8).

In the deeper layer there are the ulnar vessels and nerve *(44)*.

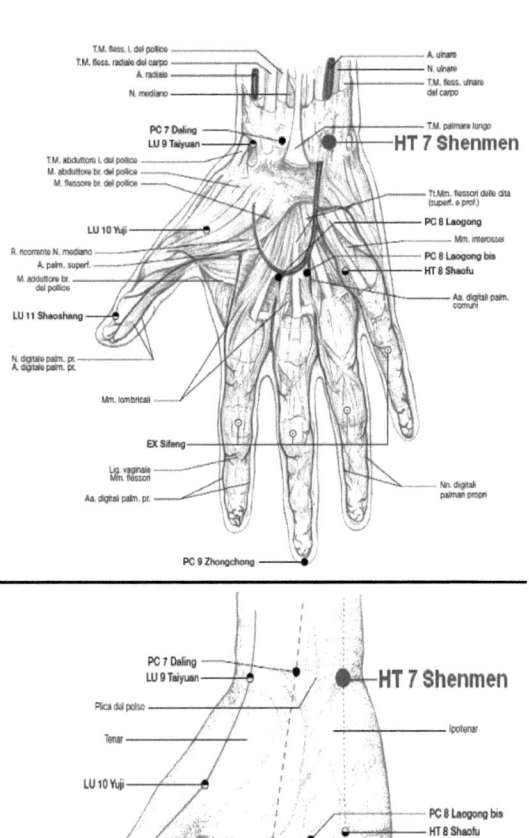

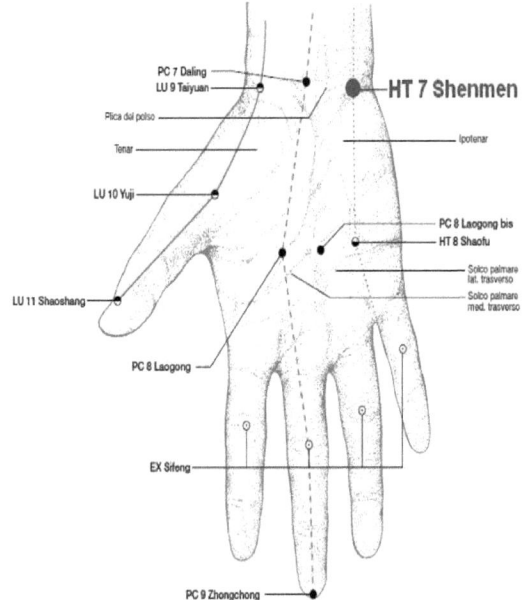

20

Comparison between clinical indications of Western medicine and Traditional Chinese Medicine

Western Medicine	Traditional Chinese Medicine
Anxiety, agitation, neurasthenia, insomnia, amnesia, palpitations, aphasia.	*Heart-Qi* and *Heart-Blood* deficiency. Calms the mind.
Pain in the ulnar aspect of wrist and hand.	*Bi* syndrome.
Chest oppression, heart pain radiated to upper limb, heart pain, arhythmia.	Stagnation of *Qi* and *Blood* or *Phlegm* in the *Heart* and in the *Heart Channel.*

Remarks: this acupoint is the most used to treat anxiety manifestations and insomnia. However its main action seems to be that of reinforcing mental abilities and self-control. Therefore it has not only a sedative effect. This point is also used to treat heart diseases.

This acupoint is the most important of *Heart Channel*. It can be used in any syndrome of *Heart* to calm the *Shen*, which is its main function. However, in the first place, it nourishes the *Heart Blood* and it is the point of choice in case of deficiency of *Heart Blood* that causes anxiety, insomnia, poor memory, palpitations and pale tongue.

In some Randomized Clinical Trials is highlighted how the acupressure of *HT7* point (*Shenmen*) improves the parameters of sleep quality: sleep latency, sleep duration, habitual sleep efficiency, and sleep disturbances in general *(45)*.

7. The efficacy of acupressure for insomnia and other sleep disorders in institutionalized elderly with dementia

Objectives :

Our study want to show that acupressure treatment is feasible also in elderly institutionalized patients suffering from Alzheimer's disease with mild cognitive impairment

and it is effective in treating of insomnia. Furthermore, the treatment with acupressure improves the quality of sleep.

We administered to patients enrolled various assessment scales (Global Deterioration Scale – GDS; Mini Mental State Examination – MMSE; Neuropsychiatric Inventory – NPI; State-Trait-Anxiety Inventory – STAI Y-1; Activity Daily Living – ADL; Instrumental Activity Daily Living – IADL; Pittsburg Sleep Quality Index – PSQI; Global Health Questionnaire – GHQ 28).

I. Mini Mental State Examination (MMSE) :

The "Mini Mental State Examination" (MMSE) is a screening test which is a rapid and sensitive tool for the exploration of cognitive functions and its changes over time and it is applicable even in severe forms of cognitive impairment.

It requires an administration time of approximately 10-15 minutes and it is divided into 30 items that assess *(46)*:

o   The space-time orientation
o   The ability to keep attention
o   The ability of learning and recall new verbal semantically unstructured material
o   The comprehension of verbal and written order, writing skill and ability to denomination
o   Praxic and constructive skill.

The overall rating is directly proportional to the efficiency of cognitive functions. The maximum value is 30. It' s necessary to correct the raw score for age and education (see table). Is considered normal a correct score greater than 24/30.

Coefficients of adjustment of MMSE by age and education in the Italian population (*Magni et al, 1996*).

EDUCATION	AGE	65-69	0-74	75-79	80-84	85-89
0-4 years		+ 0.4	+ 0.7	+ 1.0	+ 1.5	+ 2.2
5-7 years		- 1.1	- 0.7	- 0.3	+ 0.4	+ 1.4
8-12 years		- 2.0	- 1.6	- 1.0	- 0.3	+ 0.8
13-17 years		- 2.8	- 2.3	- 1.7	- 0.9	+ 0.3

The MMSE is effective as a screening tool able to separate patients with cognitive impairment from those without it. In addition, when it's used repeatedly the instrument is able to measure changes in cognitive status after therapeutic intervention.

However, this tool is based heavily on verbal response and on reading and writing abilities. Therefore, patients that are hearing and visually impaired or that have low literacy or those with other communication disorders may perform poorly even if cognitively intact.

II.   Global Deterioration Scale (GDS) :

The most common scale for staging Alzheimer's disease is the Global Deterioration Scale (GDS). This scale is a tool for comprehensive assessment of severity of cognitive impairment and it is designed to monitor over time the progression of Alzheimer's disease.

The GDS is a 7-level scale of severity of cognitive impairment (from "no decline" to "severe dementia").

The Global Deterioration Scale (GDS), developed by Dr. Barry Reisberg, provides an overview on stages of cognitive functions in patients suffering from a primary degenerative dementia such as Alzheimer's disease. It is divided into 7 different stages. Stages 1-3 are considered pre-dementia stages. Stages 4-7 are "dementia stages". Beginning in stage 5, a patient cannot survive longer without assistance.

STAGE 1 – Subjectively and objectively normal

STAGE 2 – Very mild cognitive impairment : subjective complaints of mild memory loss; objectively normal on testing; no functional deficit.

STAGE 3 – Mild Congnitive Impairment (MCI) : earliest clear-cut deficits; functionally normal but co-workers may be aware of declining work performance; objective deficits on testing; denial may appear.

STAGE 4 – Early dementia: evidence of clear deficits in a careful clinical interview; difficulty to perform complex tasks, e.g. handling finances, travelling; denial behaviors and difficulties in challenging situations are common.

STAGE 5 – Moderate dementia :   patients can no longer survive without assistance; they are unable to recall major and relevant aspects of their current lives, e.g. an adress or a telephone number,the names of grandchildren...; there can be some temporal disorientation (difficulties to remember the correct day of the week or the current season) or some difficulties to place; they require no assistance in toileting, eating or dressing but they may need help to choose appropriate clothings.

STAGE 6 – Moderate-severe dementia: patients may occasionally forget name of spouse; there can be a large unaware of recent experiences and events of their lives; they will require assistance in basic ADLs; they can suffer from urine incontinence; behavioural and psychological symptoms of dementia (BPSD) are common, e.g. delusions, repetitive behaviours, agitation.

STAGE 7 – Severe dementia : verbal abilities coud be lost in the course of this stage; patients are incontinent; they needs assistance in feeding and they can lose ability to walk *(47)*.

III. Neuropsychiatric Inventory (NPI) :

The Neuropsychiatric Inventory (NPI) allows to identify, through the information given by patients' family members, a wide range of behavioral changes and their impact on caregivers' distress. This is an interview with questions related to six weeks before. They consider the behavioral changes arising after the disease onset and they do not investigate the premorbid characteristics of the patient.

In our study, we used the 12 domains version *(48)* that has been designed for use in residential settings. Studies in literature also considered it as a useful tool for monitoring the progress of clinical BPSD and the efficacy of pharmacological interventions for their control *(49, 50)*.

Neuropsychiatric Inventory considers the following domains:

• Delusions
• Hallucinations
• Agitation
• Depression / dysphoria
• Anxiety
• Euphoria / exaltation
• Apathy / Indifference
• Disinhibition
• Irritability / lability
• Physical activity
• Sleep
• Disturbances in appetite and food intake

Any behavioral change is measured by a subjective caregiver assessment considering the frequency of the symptoms (0 - absence of symptoms and 4 – when symptoms are always present) and its severity (1 means mild symptoms that do not produce disturbances and 3 means severe and very disturbing symptoms).

The total score is calculated multiplying the frequency for the gravity for each sub-item. Every single behavioral manifestation will then have a score ranging from 0 to 12.

Subsequently the final score is calculated by adding up the individual scores. There will be an overall score which can range from 0 (no behavioral problems) to 144 (high presence and severity of behavioral disorders).

You can also assess the burden of care perceived by the primary caregiver. These data do not enter in the calculation of the final score but it provides an assessment of how the behavioral disorders affect psychological and emotional aspects of caregivers. Also in this case an opinion on the emotional and psychological stress perceived is asked to the caregiver. This one provides a rating from 0 (absence of emotional and psychological stress) to 5 (severe emotional and psychological stress). The final score may vary in a range from a minimum of 0 to a maximum of 60.

IV.   General Health Questionnaire 28 (GHQ 28) :

GHQ 28 has been developed to identify two main categories of problems: " *the inability to carry out one's normal healthy functions and the appearance of new phenomena of distressing nature" (51).* The GHQ 28 has been validated in different types of patients: patients with cerebral stroke, patients with spinal cord injury and patients with myocardial infarction *(52, 53)*.

There are several versions of this questionnaire: in our work we used the 28-item version that detects the presence and the frequency of non chronic symptoms. Each item is characterized by a description of positive psychological states and of activities of daily living (eg, the ability to concentrate, feeling useful, ..) but also of negative symptoms of psychological distress (eg, loss of sleep, inability to overcome the difficulties ...). The patient must assess the presence and the frequency of symptoms (those are not chronic) during weeks before the interview.

The items are divided into 4 steps, each one consisting of 7 items:

• Somatic symptoms;
• Anxiety and insomnia;
• Social dysfunction;
• Severe depression.

The subject is asked to compare their current situation its usual state of mind, choosing between 4 responses (for positive items: "better than usual", "as usual", "less than usual", "much less than usual "; for negative items : "no", "no more than usual", "a little more than usual", "much more than usual").

The aim of the questionnaire is to assess changes in normal psychic functioning. It does not investigate the presence of severe mental disorders such as schizophrenia or psychotic depression or of personality disorders or patterns of adaptation associated with distress.

To score the scale, in our study, we used the method "Likert" that assigns a 0-1-2-3 score for the 4 types of response and allows to obtain, within the overall score, some information about intensity and frequency of symptoms. It is possible to place individuals along a continuum from "psychological well-being", considered as the absence of psychic symptoms, to a condition of "psychic disorder" with varying degrees of severity.

V.   State Trait Anxiety Inventory Y-1 (STAY) :

The term "anxiety" is generally used to denote an emotional state characterized by a variable set of symptoms and psychological, physiological and behavioral signs closely related to each other. In particular, the anxiety is *"nervous disorder marked by excessive uneasiness and apprehension, typically with compulsive behaviour or panic attacks with a feeling of worry, nervousness, or unease about something with an uncertain outcome" (54).*

The State Trait Anxiety Inventory is a test consisting of 40 items: 20 measure the anxiety state and 20 measure the anxiety trait. The state anxiety refers to an emotional state at a clear time, whereas the anxiety trait refers to a personality characteristic. To compile the scale about state anxiety, the subject must respond to items based on how you feel at that precise moment. To compile the scale about anxiety trait, the subject must respond according to how you usually feel. In our study, we used only the scale of anxiety state (STAI-Y) consisting of 20 items that measure anxiety on a 4 levels intensity scale.

1 "for nothing"
2 "a little bit"
3 "enough"
4 "very much".

For each response of STAI-Y is assigned a weighted score from 1 to 4. The final score is obtained by summing the responses to each item: the higher the score is, the greater the level of anxiety experienced by the subject will be. The STAI-Y is a questionnaire widely used in various fields and it's a valid instrument for neuropsychological assessment *(55).*

VI.   Pittsburg Sleep Quality Index (PSQI) :

The Pittsburg Sleep Quality Index (PSQI) is a questionnaire that assesses the quality of sleep and its disorders.

The PSQI is a self-assessment scale that has been developed in order to provide a reliable, valid and standardized measure of quality of sleep and it provides a rapid, clinically useful assessment of different types of sleep impairment.

The scale consists of 19 items that are combined in 7 parts, with a score that varies from 0 to 3.

In all cases, the score "0" indicates the absence of difficulty while the score "3", the presence of serious difficulties. The global PSQI score, which can range from 0 to 2 is obtained from the sum of the scores of the 7 components: higher scores indicate greater impairment of sleep.

These 7 items assess:

1. the subjective quality of sleep;
2. the sleep latency;
3. the sleep duration;
4. the habitual effectiveness of sleep;
5. sleep disorders in general;
6. the use of hypnotic drugs;
7. disturbances during the day.

It is a questionnaire able to identify specific disorders of sleep and it is characterized by having good psychometric properties and the presence of cut-off scores.

The PSQI shows, finally, an index of reliability (reliability coefficient Cronbach's α) of 0.835, indicating a high degree of internal consistency *(56)*.

VII.   Activity of Daily Living (ADL) :

The Activity of Daily Living (ADL) is a scale used to measure the efficacy of performances in common activities of daily living.

The index examines six variables: feeding, dressing, managing personal hygiene, bathing, move independently, continence. The score is the number of preserved functions, and it varies from 0 to 6 point. The scale is an essential tool for evaluation of physical function.

ADL is one of the most used tools in geriatric/psychogeriatric assessment as regards prognostic and preventive areas and it can assess the effects of treatments *(57)*.

VIII.   Instrumental Activity of Daily Living (IADL) :

The IADL assesses activities related to the level of independence of the elderly in the instrumental abilities of daily living. These skills are considered more complex than the basic activities of daily living as measured by the Katz Index of ADL.

The IADL are activities that allow to live independently such as the ability to use the phone, to prepare meals, to make purchases in stores, to do housework, to take drugs, to use means of transport, to do laundry and to manage the use of money.

The Lawton IADL scale measures 8 function domains. Historically, women were scored on all 8 areas of function; men were not scored in the domains of food preparation, housekeeping, laundering. However, current recommendations are to assess all domains for both genders *(58)*.

Persons are scored according to their highest level of functioning in that category. A summary score ranges from 0 (low function, dependent) to 8 (high function, independent).

Methods :

A longitudinal prospective study was used to test the efficacy and tolerability of acupressure to treat insomnia in old people, especially in those affected by dementia. Our research is conformed to The Helsinki Declaration and to our local legislation; it has been approved by our Ethic Committee (ASL TO2 Comitato Etico prot. N. 18438/13 del 3/4/2013. Titolo I categ. 2 Classe 5).

The purpose of our research was clearly explained by physicians to patients and relatives, if present, and the informed consent was collected from patients or legal guardians; privacy has been guaranteed.

The participants were recruited from two 178-bed nursing homes specialized in the care of patients affected by Alzheimer's dementia with Mild Cognitive Impairment and, in particular, by behavioral disturbances (27-beds dedicated). We enrolled 129 patients aged between 69 and 96 years (82,65 ± 7,26) suffering from both primary and secondary insomnia usually treated with sedative drugs.

Recruitment criteria were: (I) patients suffering from sleep disturbance, both primary and secondary insomnia in patients with Alzheimer's disease and Mild Cognitive Impairment; (II) patients affected by Alzheimer's disease according to NINCDS-ADRDA criteria *(59)* ; and (III) disease staging was performed with the Global Deterioration Scale *(GDS)* *(47)* and just patients with Mild Cognitive Impairment (*MCI*) (level 0 to 3) were enrolled.

Patients suffering from severe dementia were excluded because of their inability to pay attention for a long time and consequently to perform the tests.

The correct practice of manual HT7 point (*Shenmen*) acupressure requires a constant pressure that has to be maintained for an appropriate time. This stimulation can be realized using special plastic "pressing buttons", characterized by an easy application and a good stimulation of the point.

The device *H7 Insomnia Control®* consists of a small, smooth, soft and plastic button fixed to a patch, that can create and maintain a calibrated pressure on the HT7 point in both wrists, reproducing the benefits of manual acupressure.

The pressure can be applied locally for a certain period of time (at least 15 – 30'), or applied pressing a button at the center of the point and then stop it firmly superimposing an adhesive plaster.

So, we have applied *H7 Insomnia Control®* for 8 h. A constant pressure is ensured by an adhesive patch put on the button and it is maintained in the correct site for all night long (from 7 pm to 7 am).

The nursing staff and the care workers (39 care workers participated in the application of the study protocol) has been instructed to the correct administration and removal of the device by physicians. The location of the HT7 (*Shenmen*) point is the following: on the skin crease of the wrist, between the pisiform bone and the ulna, in the medial depression of the tendon of ulna flexor muscle of the wrist.

To correctly locate this acupoint you can proceed as follows **(Fig.1)** :

1) bend your hand slightly, in order to highlight the thin line that, at its base, separates it from the forearm,

2) divide this line into two equal parts by a line A,

3) divide to two further parts the outer half (on the side of the little finger) with a line B,

4) at the intersection between the line B and the fold of wrist flexion, corresponding to a pit located within a tendon, there is HT 7 point (*Shenmen*) *(60)*.

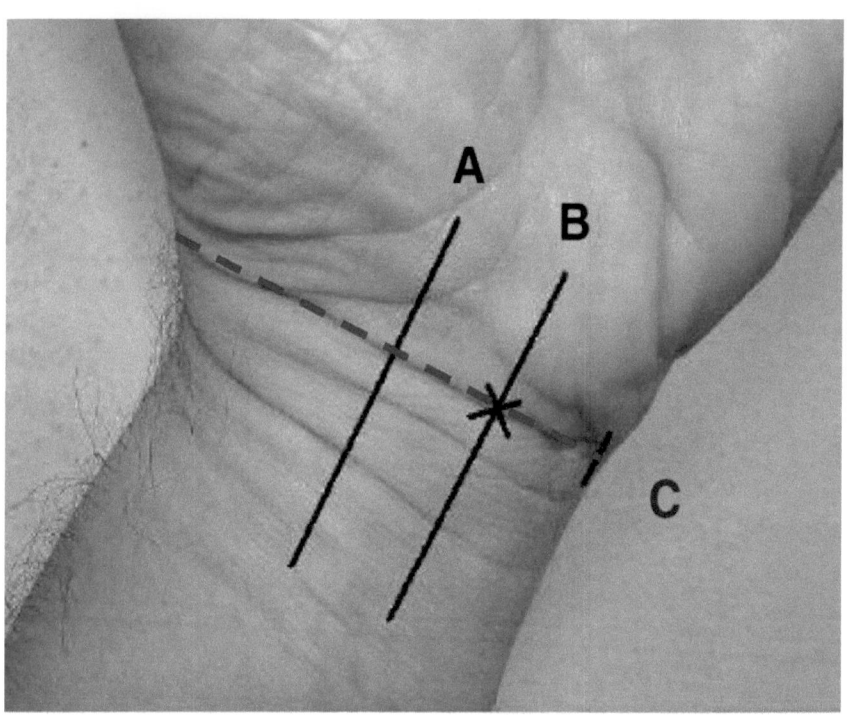

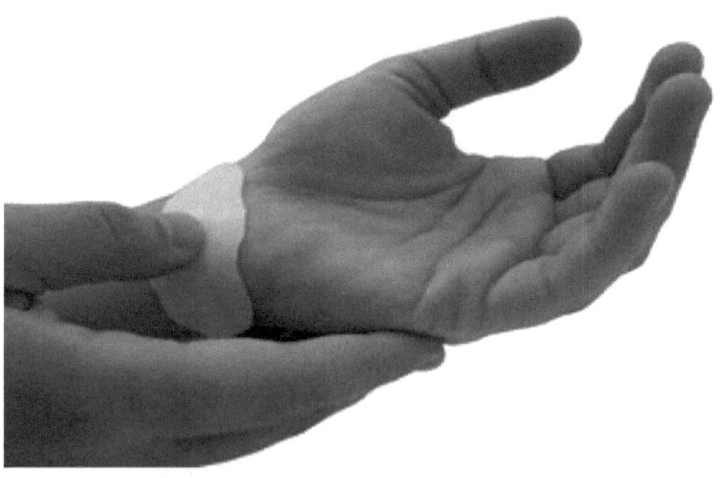

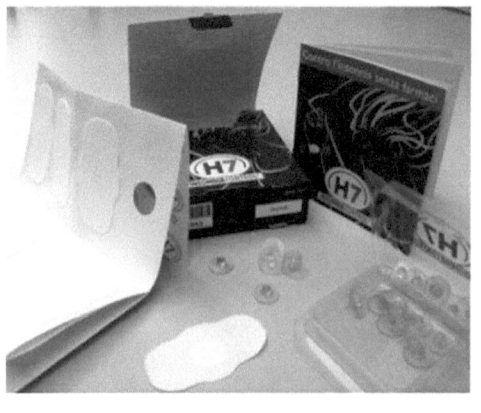

Fig. 1 *Correct location of acupoint HT7 (Shenmen) Line A divides the blue thin line C that separates the hand from the forearm into two equal parts. Line B divides to two further parts the outer half (on the side of the little finger). HT7 is the crossing between line C and line B (61, 62, 63).*

The *H7 Insomnia Control®* device has been applied every evening 30 minutes before sleep by the nursing staff and removed by care workers the following morning during the daily care, so the HT 7 point (*Shenmen*) stimulation lasted constantly all night long. The treatment lasted 2 months.

At first, anamnestic and clinical data of all the enrolled patients have been performed, involving caregiver and nursing staff. Particular attention has been paid to the use of sedative drugs.

At the beginning of the study (T0), for the cognitive and behavioral assessment we gave to patients the Mini Mental State Examination (MMSE) *(46)*, the Global Deterioration Scale (GDS) *(47)*, the Neuropsychiatric Inventory (NPI) *(48)* and the State-Trait-Anxiety Inventory (STAI Y-1) *(55)*; for the evaluation of the functional state we gave the Activity Daily Living (ADL) and the Instrumental Activity Daily Living (IADL) according to Katz and Lawton *(57, 58)*.

Besides, the Global Health Quality of Life (GHQ 28) *(51, 52, 53)*, (including these four aspects: health, mood, social activities, metacognitive sphere) and the Pittsburgh Sleep Quality Index (PSQI) *(56)*, based on subjective opinion of the quality of sleep, were also administrated. The same measurements were carried out after 2 months - at the end of the treatment (T1) - and 4 months after the end of treatment (T2).

At last, if a patient at T1 or T2 could not perform tests because of communication problems, due to a rapid progress of his/her disease, the evaluation was limited to the NPI. The NPI was administered to the caregiver, following the same temporal criteria: T0 , T1 and T2, but these data were not included in the statistics, in order to avoid confounding factors. For statistical analysis we used SPSS Statistical Package for the Social Sciences, SPSS, Release 17 *(SPSS Inc., Chicago, IL , 2009)* and it was conducted with ANOVA.

Results :

PSQI was significantly correlated to the GHQ28 ($p = 0,003$), showing how the feeling of a good sleep quality encourages the perception of a better general health status ($p < 0,001$).

GHQ28 detected also a statistically positive difference in particular in section B, as concerning sleep and mood ($p < 0,001$) **(Fig. 2)**

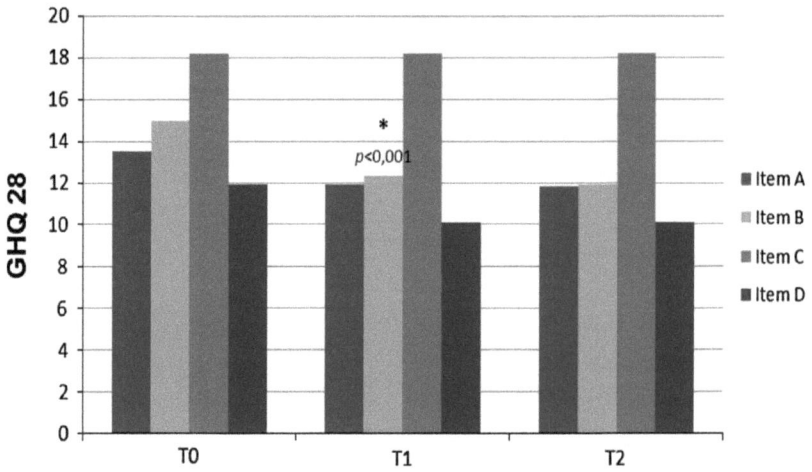

Fig. 2 *GHQ28 (Global Health Quality of Life) divided by items explored at T0, T1, and T2 items:* ***a.*** *somatic symptoms;* ***b.*** *mood (anxiety/insomnia);* ***c.*** *social dysfunction;* ***d.*** *severe depression GHQ28 detected a statistically positive difference in particular in section B as concerning sleep and mood ($p < 0.001$).*

Instead the perception of sleep (PSQI) highlighted an important positive answer at T1 (after 1 month) (*p < 0,001*) and it was maintained at T2 (after 4 months) (*p = 0,005*). In particular, PSQI detected that the number of hours of effective sleep, was perceived as increased at T1 in every patient, with an average of slept hours between 5 and 7 every night (**Fig. 3**).

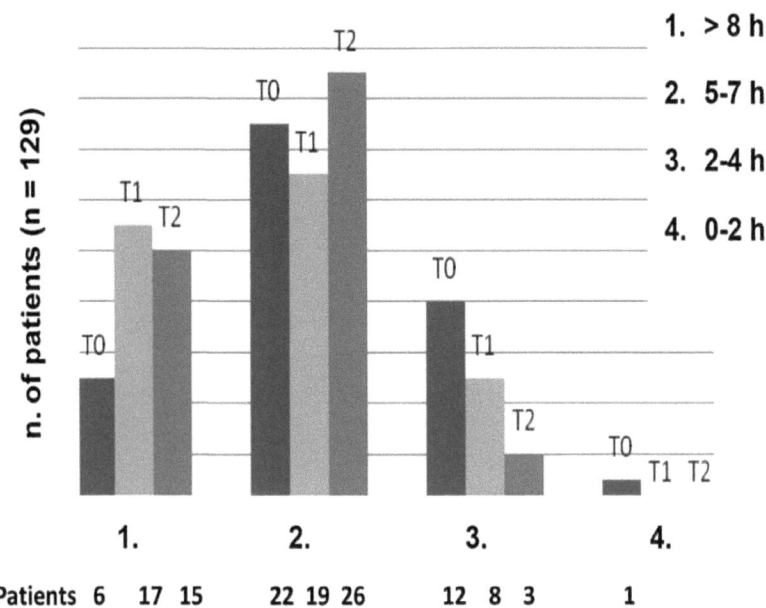

Patients   6   17   15   22   19   26   12   8   3   1

Fig. 3 Hours of sleep measured by PSQI (Pittsburg sleep quality index) at T0, T1, and T2. The perception of sleep (PSQI) highlighted an important positive answer at T1 (p < 0.001) and it was maintained at T2 (p = 0.005). In particular, PSQI detected that the number of
hours of effective sleep, was perceived as increased at T1 in every patient, with an average of slept hours between 5 and 7 every night.

Furthermore, in most patients, the time necessary to fall asleep decreased significantly (**Fig. 4**) and also the perceived quality of sleep increased in all patients.

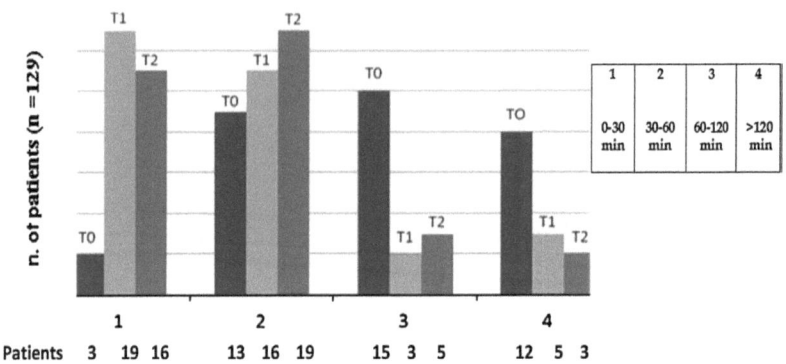

Fig. 4 *Time to fall asleep in minutes detected by PSQI (Pittsburg sleep quality index) at T0, T1 and T2. In most patients the time necessary to fall asleep decreased significantly from T0 to T1.*

Data value of NPI at T0 and at T1 showed a statistical positive correlation (12.5 ± 1.4 vs. 6.9 ± 0.7 $p < 0,001$) and this trend was maintained for the entire duration of the study (T2: 6.19 ± 0.8 vs. 6.9 ± 0.7) (**Fig. 5**). The retention index was about 97% (4 patients were excluded because of poor compliance).

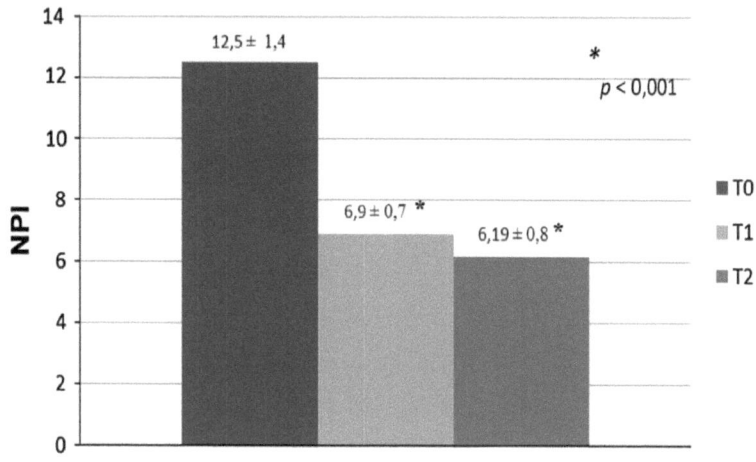

Fig. 5 *NPI (Neuropsychiatric Inventory) measured at T0, T1, and T2.*
Data value of NPI at T0 and at T1 showed a statistical positive correlation
(12.5 ± 1.4 vs. 6.9 ± 0.7 p < 0.001) and this trend was maintained for the entire
duration of the study.

Moreover, sedative drugs have been reduced in all patients involved in the study, and even in two people the administration has been stopped. STAI Y-1, both at T1 and at T2, showed a positive trend of improvement, but with a not significant difference ($p = 0,21$), probably because anxious trait was not the dominating symptom in these patients. There were not important changes in the cognitive (*MMSE*) and in the functional status (*ADL, IADL*) (**Table 1**).

No side effects were detected using acupressure.

Table 1 Variables measured at T0, T1, and T2

Variables	T0 mean (DS)	T1 mean (DS)	T2 mean (DS)	p^{**}
ADL	2 (1)	2 (1)	2 (1)	0.92
IADL	2.4 (1.1)	2.3 (1.2)	2.3 (1.2)	0.93
MMSE	18.0 (4.6)	19.8 (4.4)	18.8 (3.6)	0.38
GHQ-28	15.1 (3.9)	12.8 (3.7)	11.9 (2.8)	0.003**
PSQI	12.59 (8.56)	8.56 (3.27)	9.2 (3.6)	0.002**
NPI	12.5 (1.4)	6.9 (0.7)	6.19 (0.8)	<0.001**
STAI Y-1	78.9 (3.6)	74.6 (3.7)	74.3 (2.9)	0.21
Sedative drugs (BDZ)	3 (0.8)	2 (0.3)	1 (0.9)	<0.001**

Table 1. *ADL activity daily living, IADL instrumental activity daily living, MMSE mini mental state examination, GHQ global health quality of life, PSQI Pittsburgh sleep quality index, NPI neuropsychiatric inventory, STAI Y-1 state-trait-anxiety inventory.*

Discussion :

HT7 point (*Shenmen*) acupressure is a simple and nonintrusive therapeutic method and this study validates its efficacy in managing sleep disturbances and insomnia, bettering an important care problem in older people and improving their quality of life. Our study demonstrated the effectiveness of HT7 point (*Shenmen*) continuous nocturne acupressure in elderly institutionalized patients.

In fact, there were a reduction of sleep disturbances, an increase of effective slept hours, a much quicker sleep induction, and a better global sleep quality. The study highlighted also an positive impact on the perception of general health state and mood.

Besides, also the number of sedative drugs was importantly reduced. In our opinion, the strength of our acupressure protocol has been the continuous stimulation realized through the application of nonintrusive ''pressing buttons,'' characterized also by a practical use. In this way, we had good therapeutic results using a little time to care and supporting lower costs.

Besides, this device is not a drug and, therefore, it can also be applied safely by caregivers or patients themselves. So, the simple, easily reproducible methodology of this intervention can lead to positive outcomes as a potential, nonpharmacologic, integrated treatment in the behavioral disorders related to dementia, pursuing effectiveness, and therapeutic safety, improving these patients' health and quality of life.

A limitation of the study is the small sample size. More studies are needed to further validate the results of our study.

As previously mentioned, the study conducted by Chen et al. *(64)* demonstrated that HT7 point (*Shenmen*) acupressure improves sleep quality (measured with PSQI) in elderly institutionalized patients treated with real acupressure. Instead, the two control groups - the not treated one and the other one treated with false acupressure - did not have this benefit on sleep. Besides, in the group treated with real HT7 point (*Shenmen*) acupressure, the time of permanence in bed increased, while the number of nocturne awakening decreased. Similar results are present in a recent RCT *(65)*.

Moreover, Yang *(20)* demonstrated that subjects affected by dementia reduced their behavioral disturbances if treated with acupressure 15 min every day for a month, and these results were confirmed with a recent cross-over trial conducted by an integrated methodology between a non-pharmacological approach and an acupressure protocol *(21)*.

Also, in our study a remarkable and persistent reduction of sleep-wake rhythm alteration comes out at NPI, taking into account, in this way, the presence of other important psychotic and behavioral disturbances related to the cognitive deterioration of these patients, with a consequent reduction of nursing staff stress. Besides, persistence of the positive effect, highlighted at the follow up and present until the end of the study, is remarkable. Perhaps, this aspect is the most important because the treatment with HT7 point (*Shenmen*) acupressure could also be recommended as an efficacious and a non-intrusive method in order to decrease agitated behaviors in patients with dementia. This fact could importantly influence the course of the disease and also the quality of care.

Indeed, an effective intervention for caregivers to manage agitated behaviors could potentially save a great deal of medical costs and also many underestimated informal costs. For this reason, a further and extended research (Randomized Clinical Trial) is already in course, in order to test a possibility of an integrated intervention with TCM on an elderly population affected by insomnia and other psycho-behavioral diseases, where a real acupuncture would be too difficult to manage.

Conclusions :

Also our scientific work has confirmed the indications of acupuncture in the treatment of insomnia and in particular the use of *HT7* point, that is the most frequently used in treatment protocols.

According to the experimental results exposed, the overall assessment on the use of acupressure on *HT7* point must be considered positive.

Therefore, in light of the obtained data, it is possible to summarize the results in these following points:

- the device, *HT7 Insomnia Control* © has proven to have a positive effect on patients with insomnia;

- the use of acupressure on *HT7* is able to improve the general feeling of wellbeing, the subjective quality of sleep and to reduce the level of anxiety.

All this has a considerable impact on individual quality of life both for the improvement of subjective and objective symptoms and because of the effect achieved by the use of a minimally invasive technique and without the use of drugs.

Further studies are also needed to implement the use of Complementary Medicine such as Acupuncture and Acupressure in the common medical practice in view of a holistic vision based on the entirety of the individual.

Conflict of interest : On behalf of all authors, the corresponding author states that there is no conflict of interest.

8.   References :

1.   Spence DW, Kayumov L, Chen A et al. *Acupuncture increases nocturnal melatonin secretion and reduces insomnia and anxiety: A preliminary report.* J Neuropsychiatry Clin Neurosci 2004; 16(1): 19-28.

2.   Park HJ et al. *The effect of acupuncture on anxiety and neuropeptide Y expression in the basolateral amygdala of maternally separated rats.* Neurosci Lett Apr 4; 377 (3): 179-184, 2005.

3.   Futaesaku Y, Zhai N, Ono M, Watanabe M, Zhao J, Zhang C, Li L, Shi X. *Brain activity of a rat reflects apparently the stimulation of acupuncture. A radioautography using 2-deoxyglucose.* Dept. of Histology and Analytical Morphology, School of Allied Health Science, Kitasato University, Kanagawa, Japan. *Cell Mol Biol (Noisy-le-grand).1995 Feb;41(1):161-70.*

4.   Kim MR, Kim SJ, Lyu YS, Kim SH, Lee Y, Kim TH, Shim I, Zhao R, Golden GT, Yang CH. *Effect of acupuncture on behavioral hyperactivity and dopamine release in the nucleus accumbens in rats sensitized to morphine.* Department of Pharmacology, College of Oriental Medicine, Daegu Haany University, Daegu 706-828, South Korea *Neurosci Lett. 2005 Oct 14;387(1):17-21.*

5.   Gooneratne NS. *Complementary and alternative medicine for sleep disturbances in older adults.* Clin Geriatr Med 2008; 24(1):121-38.

6.   Cheuk DK, Yeung WF, Chung KF et al. *Acupuncture for insomnia.* Cochrane Database Syst Rev 2007; Jul 18(3):CD005472.

7.   Wu HS, Wu SC, Lin JG et al. *Effectiveness of acupressure in improving dyspnoea in chronic obstructive pulmonary disease.* J Adv Nurs 2004; 45: 252-259.

8.   Chen M L, Lin LC, Wu SC et al. *The effectiveness of acupressure in improving the quality of sleep of institutionalized residents.* J Gerontol A Biol Sci Med Sci 1999; 54(8): M389-94.

9.   Tsay SL, Rong JR, Lin PF. *Acupoint massage in improving the quality of sleep and quality of life in patients with end-stage renal disease.* J Adv Nurs 2003; 42: 134-142.

10.   Yang MH, Lin Lc., *Acupressure in the care of the elderly.* Hu Li Za Zhi31: 54(4): 10-15, 2007.

11.   Lin LC et al., *Using acupressure and Montessori-based activities to decrease agitation for residents with dementia: a cross-over trial.* J Am Geriatr Soc 57(6): 1022-9, 2009.

12. Pavao TS et al. *Acupuncture is effective to attenuate stress and stimulate lynphocyte proliferation in the elderly.* Neurosci Lett. 2010 Oct 22;484(1):47-50.

13. Terry RD, Peck A, De Teresa R, *Some morphometric aspects of the brain in senile dementia of Alzheimer type.* Ann Neurol 10: 184-192; 1981.

14. Terry RD, Peck A, De Teresa R, *Some morphometric aspects of the brain in senile dementia of Alzheimer type.* Ann Neurol 10: 184-192; 1981.

15. Petersen RC et al. *Mild Cognitive impairment: clinical characterization and outcome.* Archives of Neurology 56, 303-308, 1999.

16. Petersen RC, et al. *Current concepts in mild cognitive impairment.* Archives of Neurology 58, 1985-1992, 2001.

17. Esiri MM, *The basis for behavioural disturbances in dementia.* J Neurol Neurosurg Psychiatry 61: 127-130, 1996.

18. Liu Hj. *Acupuncture cures disease from the relations of channels, bowels and viscera.* Liao Ning TCM 2002; 29: 70.

19. Huang L; *Clinical observations of treatment of dementia with acupuncture and massage.* New TCM 1996; 25-26.

20. Yang MH, Wu SC, Lin JG et al. *The efficacy of acupressure for decreasing agitated behaviour in dementia: a pilot study.* J Clin Nurs 2007; 16: 308–315.

21. Li-Chan L, Man-Hua Y, Chieh-Chun K et al. *Using Acupressure and Montessori- Based Activities to Decrease Agitation for Residents with Dementia: A Cross-Over Trial.* J Am Geriatr Soc 2009; 57: 1022–1029.

22. Nordio M, Romanelli F. *Efficacy of wrists overnight compression (HT 7 point) on insomniacs: possible role of melatonin?* Minerva Med 2008; 99(6): 539-47.

23. Lee SY, Baek YH, Park SU et al. *Intradermal acupuncture on shen-men and nei- kuan acupoints improves insomnia in stroke patients by reducing the sympathetic nervous activity: a randomized clinical trial.* Am J Chin Med 2009; 37(6): 1013-21.

24. Fu WB, Fan L et al. *Depressive neurosis treated bu acupuncture for regulating the liver – a report of 176 cases.* Tradit Chin Med Jun; 29 (2): 83-6, 2009.

25. Sun H et al. *Effect of acupuncture at Baihui (GV 20) and Zusanli (ST36) on the level of serum inflammatory cytochines in patients with depression.* Zhongguo Zhen Jiu Mar 30 (3): 195-9, 2010.

26. Zhang et al. *Combination of acupuncture and fluoxetine for depression: a randomized, double-blind, sham-controlled trial.* Altern Complement Med aug;15

(89): 837-44, 2009.

27. Torjesen I et al. *Adding acupuncture or counseling to usual care hastens improvement in persistent depression.* Sep 25; 347: f5789, 2013.

28. Li HJ et al. *Acupuncture for post-stroke depression: a randomized control trial.* Zhongguo Zhen Jiu Jan; 31 (1): 3-6, 2011.

29. Zheng GC et al. *Meta-analysis of the curative effect of acupuncture on post-stroke depression.* J Tradit Chin Med Mar; 32 (1): 6-11, 2012.

30. Smith CA et al. *Acupuncture for depression.* Cochrane Database Syst Rev Jan 20; (1): CD004046, 2010.

31. Zhang ZJ et al. *The effectiveness and safety of acupuncture therapy in depressive disorders: systematic review and meta-analysis.* J Affect Disord Jul; 124 (1-2): 9-21, 2010.

32. Fetveit A. *Late-life insomnia: a review.* Geriatr Gerontol Int 2009; 9: 220-234

33. Winkelman JW. *Diagnosis and treatment of insomnia.* New York, Prescribing Reference, Inc., 2005.

34. Cohen CA, Colantonio A, Vernich L. *Positive aspects of caregiving: rounding out the caregiver experience.* International Journal of Geriatric Psychiatry 2002; 17: 184 -188.

35. Balla S, Simoncini M, Giacometti I et al. *The daily center care on impact of family burden. Arch* Gerontol Geriatr 2007; 44(Suppl 1): 55-9.

36. Sarris J, Byrne GJ. *A systematic review of insomnia and complementary medicine.* Sleep Med Rev 2011; 15 (2): 99-106.

37. Cao H, Pan X, Li H, Liu J. *Acupuncture for treatment of insomnia: a systematic review of randomized controlled trials.* J Altern Complement Med 2009; 15(11): 1171-86.

38. Yeung WF et al. *Electroacupuncture for primary insomnia: a randomized control trial.* Sleep Aug 1; 32(8): 1039-1947.

39. Guo J et al. *Efficacy of acupuncture for primary insomnia: a randomized controlled clinical trial.* Evid Based Complement Alternat Med Epub Sep 18, 2013: 163850.

40. Jiang B et al. *Auricolar acupuncture for insomnia: a randomized controlled trial.* Zhonghua Liu Xing Bing Xue Za Zhi Dec 31(12): 1400-2, 2010

41. Kaptchuk TJ. *Medicina Cinese. Fondamenti e Metodo.*

42. http://lieske.com/channels/5e-heart.htm

43. Maciocia G. *Fondamenti della medicina cinese.*

44. PE Quirico, T Pedrali: Teaching Atlas of Acupuncture, Thieme, Stuggard New York, 2007

45. Reza H, Kian N, Pouresmail Z, Masood K, Sadat Seyed Bagher M, Cheraghi MA. *The effect of acupressure on quality of sleep in Iranian elderly nursing home residents.* Complement Ther Clin Pract 2010; 16 (2): 81-5.

46. Folstein MF, Folstein SE, McHugh PR. *Mini-mental state: a pratical method for grading the cognitive state of patients for the clinician.* Journal of Psychiatric Research 1975; 12: 189-198.

47. Reisberg B, Ferris Sh, de Leon MY et al. *Global Deterioration Scale (GDS).* Psychofarmacol Bull 1988; 24: 661- 663.

48. Cummings JL, Mega M, Gray K et al. *Neuropsychiatric Inventory (NPI)* Neurology 1994; 44: 2308-2314.

49. Zuidema SU, de Jonghe JF, Verhey FR, Koopmans RT. *Neuropsychiatric symptoms in nursing home patients: factor structure invariance of the Dutch nursing home version of the neuropsychiatric inventory in different stages of dementia..* Dement Geriatr Cogn Disord. 2007;24(3):169-76. Epub 2007 Jul 17.

50. Aalten P, De Vugt ME, Jaspers N, Jolles J, Verhey FRJ.*The course of neuropsychiatric symptoms in dementia. Part I: findings from the two-year longitudinal Maasbed study.* Int J Geriatr Psychiatry 2005; 20: 523-530

51. Goldberg DP, Hillier VF. *A scaled version of the General Health Questionnaire.* Psychol Med 1979;9:139-45.

52. Goldberg D, Gater R, Sartorius N et al. *The validity of two versions of the G.H.Q. in the WHO study of mental illness in general health care.* Psychological Medicine 1997; 27: 191-197.

53. Goldberg DP, Oldehinkel T, Ormel J. *Why GHQ threshold varies from one place to another.* Psychol Med 1998; 28(4): 915-2.

54. http://www.oxforddictionaries.com

55. Spielberger CD, Gorsuch RL, Lushene PR et al. *Manual for the State-Trait Anxiety Inventory (Form Y).* Consulting Psychologists Press Inc, Palo Alto. 1983.

56. Buysse, DJ, Reynolds CF, Monk TH et al. *The Pittsburgh Sleep Quality Index (PSQI): A new instrument for psychiatric research and practice.* Psychiatry Research 1989; 28:193-213.

57.   Katz S, Downs TD, Cash HR, Grotz RC. *Progress in development of the index of   ADL.* Gerontologist 1970; 10(1):20-30.

58.   Lawton MP, Brody EM. *Assessment of older people: self-maintaining and instrumental activities of daily living.* Gerontologist 1969; 9:179-186.

59.   McKhann G, Drachman D, Folstein M et al. *Clinical diagnosis of Alzheimer's disease: report of the NINCDS-ADRDA Work Group under the auspices   of Department of Health and   Human   Services Task Force on Alzheimer's Disease.* Neurology 1984; 34(7): 939-44.

60.   Quirico PE, Pedrali T. *Teaching Atlas of Acupuncture. Channels and Points. 2007, Vol 1.* Thieme, New York.

61.   http://www.h7insomniacontrol.ch/prodotto.php

62.   http://www.ebvertrieb.de/index.php?option=com_content&task=view&id=47&Itemid=66

63.   http://www.consulteamsas.com/h7_cosa.htm

64.   Chen M L, Lin LC, Wu SC et al. *The effectiveness of acupressure in improving the quality of sleep of institutionalized residents.* J Gerontol A Biol Sci Med Sci 1999; 54(8): M389-94.

65.   Sun JL, Sung MS, Huang MY et al. *Effectiveness of acupressure for residents of long-term care facilities with insomnia: a randomized controlled trial.* Int J Nurs Stud. 2010; 47(7): 798-805.

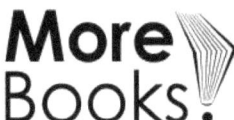
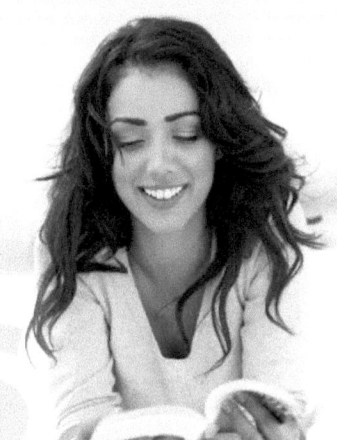
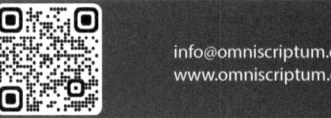
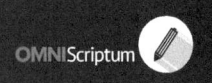

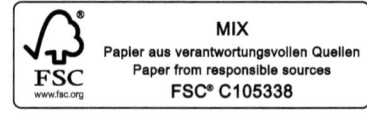